E.A. KELLER

How to Keep Your Child Healthy From Spring to Spring

A Mother Tips and Tricks To Raising Resilient Children

"It is not how much you do, but how much love you put into the doing that matters."

~MOTHER TERESA

Contents

One

Chapter 1 Welcome!

Welcome!

Hey everyone! It's great to have you here. I'm excited to share some wonderful experiences and insights I've gained over the years of living and parenting. I come from a long line of large families, and it's been quite a journey. I'm a proud mom of 10 children, and let me tell you, life's had its fair share of ups and downs.

The learning curve began back in 2006 when my first child was born. Feeding struggles led us to formula, but amidst the challenges, there were some wonderful milestones. She met growth benchmarks and became my first teacher in this parenting adventure. My son followed, making parenting seem like a breeze with his great sleep habits and easy potty training. His peaceful and happy-go-lucky personality added joy to our family.

Then came my angel baby girl, a happy and easy-going child who needed nothing more than a bit of guidance to be a happy kid. Life took unexpected turns, and I found myself divorced from the father of my first three children. After a few years, fate led me to my current husband, who brought his two beautiful daughters into our lives. Our union created a blended family of seven, and over the years, we added five more children to our beautiful family. Challenges came with those years, my two younger sons needed hospital care within the first few months of being born, I also had three of my children needing jaundice care after birth, and I also had babies who were a breeze to raise! So many ups and downs involved with parenting and child-rearing.

One thing I've learned also along the way; if it works for a child then it will work for an adult! I've shared these tips with my kids' grandparents and great-grandparents, and all have been helpful to those who try them!

In essence, my purpose in weaving these experiences is to share the lessons learned on this roller coaster of life, hoping to inspire and assist others in their unique parenting journeys. It's about embracing the complexities, finding joy in the simple moments, and creating a harmonious blended family that thrives despite life's ups and downs.

Inspiration for this book:

The idea for this book stems from my life experiences and the wish to share some straightforward insights and tips. Through my journey, I've learned not just how to foster a happy family, but more importantly, how to cultivate a healthy one. As I approach the later stages of life, where imparting parenting wisdom becomes a part of my role, I feel the urge to document this learning in real-time. The inspiration is grounded in my kids, and my aspiration to raise healthy, polite, and capable individuals.

In today's world, there are countless external influences that can impact our children in many ways. I hope to equip them with both grand and simple moments, like the kindness they show to a dog or the simple act of holding their baby sister's hand. The differences between when you truly see a person and what they shine in! Life is a blend of sweetness derived from these diverse and God-given experiences.

Two

Chapter 2 Building a Strong Foundation

Building Strong foundations

The Immune System:

Our immune system, is a marvel crafted by God, intricately designed yet surprisingly robust. It encompasses our external defenses—ears, eyes, nose, mouth—all gateways into our being. However, its primary cultivation occurs in the gut, often referred to as the microbiome or our second brain. During a natural birth, a baby receives a crucial inoculation from the mother's immune system, a vital boost for the years of life until the baby's immune system can stand on its own. While vaginal birth is optimal, we acknowledge that health considerations sometimes lead to cesarean births. Fortunately, there are ways to nurture a child's immune system in such cases, with breastfeeding playing a pivotal role. Breast milk contains unique enzymes absent in formula, despite attempts to replicate them. My personal journey attests to the varied paths of feeding, having faced the need for formula despite earnest attempts at breastfeeding. Ultimately, the key is ensuring the baby is nourished, irrespective of the method, for the best start towards a healthy child.

The Basics of A child's Immune System:

Your kiddo's immune system is like their superhero shield, keeping away all the sneaky invaders from the outside world. These can be germs like bacteria, viruses, or fungi. Think of it as a team effort involving various organs, cells, and proteins, all working together to keep your little one safe and sound. Just like a parent's watchful eye, the immune system is always on duty!

Let's break it down: your child's immune system has two main squads.

1. **The Innate Immune System:** Think of this as the superhero team your little one is born with – ready to tackle anything from day one. Think of the natural inoculation a baby receives at birth. Think of it as the rapid-response crew. It's the first to jump into action when there's a troublemaker. The team members include the skin, the eye's cornea, and the mucous membrane in the nose, tummy, and down there. They form a front line defense, protecting your little one from nasty germs, parasites, and even rogue cells like cancer. This team is like a family heirloom – passed on and ready to go from the get-go. As soon as it spots an intruder, it's all hands on deck. The immune system cells surround and take down

the invader – it's like a superhero showdown!

2. **The Acquired Immune System:** Now, this is like their growth spurt team. It kicks into action when the body meets microbes, germs, and pathogens. This crew works hand in hand with the innate team. It's like the personalized bodyguard service, creating antibodies to tackle specific troublemakers. These antibodies, crafted by B lymphocytes, stick around in your child's body, becoming their immune memory. It might take a bit for these antibodies to form, but once the immune system has faced an intruder once, it remembers and gears up for round two. It's like your child's immune system goes through superhero training, making sure they're ready to tackle any nasty bugs that come their way.

And guess what? These two teams work together – working hand in hand to keep your child Healthy and full of life.

Both teams, the rapid responders and the personalized bodyguards, are made in different body hangouts – like the adenoids in the nose, the bone marrow, lymph nodes scattered all over, lymphatic vessels, Peyer's patches in the small intestine, the spleen in the belly, the thymus behind the breastbone, and the tonsils at the back of the throat. So, you see, your kiddo's got this superhero defense league scattered all over their body, ready to take on anything that comes their way!

Tips for boosting and supporting a child's immune system:

Supplements:

Okay, let's be honest– sometimes, taking supplements can give your immune system a little extra support. But you know what's usually the star of the show? Good old food. Most of the time, getting the good stuff straight from your meals is the way to go.

Now, we totally get it – for those picky eaters or the little ones who are still figuring out their taste buds, supplements can be like a backup plan. It's a bit of extra help to make sure they're getting all the good stuff they need, especially on days when mealtime is a bit of a challenge. Just a little boost to keep everyone covered!

Remember Vitamin D!

Vitamin D = sunshine's best friend! Whenever possible, soaking in some sun is the way to go, although we know it's not always doable, especially with sunscreen and during winter.

Vitamin D-rich foods. The thing is, kids might not be in love with fatty fish or mushrooms – they're not the usual found in kid-friendly meals. But here's the scoop – you can find Vitamin D in fortified foods like milk, orange juice, yogurt, and other milk alternatives.

Oh, and here's a little tip: Vitamin D is like a tag-along with fats, so it's absorbed better when paired with some fat. Think milk with added Vitamin D, where the fat in the milk plays matchmaker. Or even in omega-three oils – they're like the perfect partners for a Vitamin D absorption party! Just a little something to keep in mind for our sunshine nutrient.

If you're thinking about Vitamin D supplements, there are plenty of options out there. It's like a whole aisle of choices – just go ahead and explore until you find one that suits you! It's all about finding what feels right for you. I've used a few a time or two during the winter myself! Some will work for you and some will work for others, which is why it's important to find one that is best for your needs.

Nuts and Seeds:

Let's talk about a powerhouse called Alpha-linolenic acid (ALA), the plant version of omega-3 fatty acids. This little hero is known to be a warrior against illnesses. Now, where can you find this goodness? Check out these top-notch sources:

- Walnuts.
- Pumpkin seeds.
- Hemp seeds.
- Chia seeds.
- Ground flax seeds.

Along with ALA these are also packed with a bunch of nutrients. We're talking protein, fiber, those "good" fats like mono- and polyunsaturated fats, plus a load of other goodies like potassium, magnesium, zinc, copper, manganese, and a lineup of vitamins – E, B6, B12, and A. It's like a nutrient treasure trove!

Fruits and Vegetables:

Here are some trusty go-tos that might sound basic, but are always winners. Fruits and veggies are like the unsung heroes, loaded with antioxidants that do wonders in protecting our cells from all kinds of trouble.

Check out these antioxidant-rich champs:

- Berries.
- Green veggies, think broccoli.
- Dark, leafy greens – we're talking spinach, kale, collard greens, and mustard greens.

Now, these power-packed foods aren't just good for the soul; they're like a nutrient goldmine. They bring in a troop of vitamins and nutrients – A, C, E, B2, B6, K, potassium, folate, magnesium, and zinc. Yep, it's a whole lot of goodness!

And here's the citrusy cherry on top – vitamin C. It's the immune-boosting rockstar, hanging out in oranges, lemons, limes, grapefruit, and let's not forget the delightful strawberries. These fruits aren't just tasty; they're like a vitamin C party waiting to happen!

Sleep and activity

First up, the magic of sleep. Good sleep is like the secret sauce for a child's immune system. So, make sure they catch those Z's – it's essential!

Below is a general rule for the best sleep amounts for children from ages 0-18;

- Infants (four to 12 months) should aim for 12 to 16 hours in a 24-hour period, naps included.
- Toddlers (one to two years) can recharge with 11 to 14 hours within 24 hours, including those daytime naps.
- Preschoolers (three to five years) should aim for 10 to 13 hours of sleep in a 24-hour cycle, naps included.
- School-age kids (six to 12 years) thrive with a good night's sleep ranging from nine to 12 hours in a 24-hour span.
- Teenagers (13 to 18 years) need their rest too, shooting for eight to 10 hours in a 24-hour period.

Activity and movement, get those little movers and shakers up and about! Regular activity isn't just a mood booster; it's a proven immunity enhancer. So, let them stretch those legs and have some fun!

Creating a conducive environment for overall well-being:
It's all about embracing the basics and fostering a healthy lifestyle across all ages. While I've shared specific tips for different age groups, these principles are universally beneficial. The key lies in crafting a well-rounded routine that encompasses everything from sleep and wake times to meals, play, moments of calm, naps, rest, education, crafting, and everything in between.

One principle I hold dear is beginning my tomorrow at 3 PM the day before. This involves planning a wholesome supper, ensuring my children follow a calming bedtime routine, and tucking them in at a reasonable hour for their bodies to rejuvenate. When they wake up the next morning having had the right amount of sleep, it sets the tone for a cheerful and vibrant day ahead.

Preparation is vital, especially for those with larger or busy families. Planning ahead, moderating sugar intake, and minimizing screen time before bedtime are small yet impactful steps that contribute to a robust immune system. It's a constant effort, and I understand it can be challenging for families with various commitments. But, remembering that a good day starts the day before, particularly around 3 PM, can guide us in making choices that prioritize afternoon snacks, nourishing dinners, and minimizing sugar and screen time before bedtime.

Additionally, having a sit-down family meal at least once a day is a practice I cherish. Whether it's breakfast in the morning or dinner in the evening, it fosters a sense of unity within the family, contributing to overall well-being. It's all about creating a routine that works for your family's unique dynamics.

Three

Chapter 3 The Power of a Nutrition

The Power of Nutrition; A. Nutrient-Rich Diet

The next factor is making sure you provide a very nutrient-rich diet. This can be difficult with picky eaters, this can be easy with kids who are happy to try lots of things. Something I like to make sure I do when it comes to introducing new foods to my kids is I always give them the choice and I try to make them try it as often as possible, even if all they do is lick it, so they get the flavor. That's easier said than done. I've definitely got a couple of picky eaters in my children and I also have kids that are happy to try anything and sometimes they trade.

It's just good to be balanced about all you do making sure that you're trying new things, introducing kids to foods at appropriate times when they're little but also just making sure it sounds fun to them and making sure that they have the choice to cause a lot of times if they don't feel like they have a choice and a situation. They'll dig their heels in really hard and they don't wanna do anything simply because you're saying they have to; so a good balance in that area, I try to have a jovial attitude about it and also a firm attitude as well. Kids thrive on boundaries. They thrive on rules even though they don't act like it.

As far as those picky eaters, one thing I like to do in a lot of the foods that I create is I will add vegetables into all of my soups. I like to cook them down real soft, not too soft, but then I like to put them in my blender and blend them up and then those vegetables become part of the broth and so you get your broth in your soup With your noodles and your meat; they don't realize that those carrots and onions and garlic is also in that broth. It's just part of the flavor.

Something else I like to do; is my kids absolutely love macaroni & cheese and I love to add carrots to my mac & cheese simply because they are the same color as the cheese sauce. So I'll warm them up and then I'll put them in my blender and then I'll add two or three tablespoons, maybe half a cup of carrots into my box of mac & cheese sauce, and that gets those veggies in that meal too.

Those are just some things you can do, simple as it sounds! You can explore it and get creative about it. You know a lot of times with casseroles, you can mix a lot of veggies in there and I find that blending them up is the best way for me because I've got some of my family who just don't like the look of the bigger veggie chunks but if I blend it up then it's no big deal they just eat the whole meal, another thing you can cook your rice or your noodles with broth, vegetable broth or beef broth or chicken broth that will add some nutrients into their meal as well.

Four

Chapter 4 The Art of Quality Sleep

The Art of Quality Sleep

Adequate sleep is a fundamental element for the mental and physical well-being of your child. However, if you're facing challenges in ensuring your toddler gets quality sleep, you're certainly not alone. According to the American Academy of Pediatrics, sleep issues impact 25 to 50 percent of children and 40 percent of adolescents.

The initial step in addressing this challenge involves understanding your child's specific sleep requirements. By incorporating good sleep hygiene practices, establishing age-appropriate routines, and being vigilant about potential sleep disorders, you can play a pivotal role in ensuring your child receives the necessary rest to thrive both physically and mentally.

Story Time! My oldest child has a terrible time sleeping and lying down to rest as a younger child around the ages of 5-8.

It was a long road to get her the proper sleep help she needed and now today she's a well-rounded almost adult! Another of my children is a night owl, she comes alive at bedtime and has a terrible time wanting to sleep, now once she's asleep, she sleeps well! Another of my children has nighttime anxiety which has proven a challenge for us. With all my children, the steps outlined next helped to guide what was the best step for each individual child!

The significance of sleep in children's lives cannot be overstated. It plays a pivotal role in the development of young minds, exerting a direct influence on happiness. Research indicates that sleep profoundly affects alertness, attention, cognitive performance, mood, resiliency, vocabulary acquisition, and the processes of learning and memory. Notably, in toddlers, napping is essential for memory consolidation, executive attention, and the development of motor skills. Additionally, sleep significantly influences growth, particularly during the early stages of infancy

Ensuring your child gets a full night's sleep involves adapting to their changing sleep needs. Regardless of age, whether dealing with a 2-year-old or a resistant teenager, research highlights the effectiveness of a consistent bedtime routine. It's beneficial to follow the same activities in the same order every day, providing a sense of predictability for your child.

A typical bedtime routine may involve:

- Turning off computers, TV screens, video games, and other bright lights
- Putting on pajamas and brushing your teeth
- Engaging in a calming activity like reading a light book,

singing a lullaby, or taking a bath
- Allowing toddlers to choose a stuffed animal or security blanket for the night

It's essential to put your child to bed when they're sleepy, not already asleep, to encourage them to learn how to fall asleep independently. For preschoolers waking up at night, gently guide them back to their bed. Avoid co-sleeping with infants, as it increases the risk of sudden infant death syndrome.

Establishing a bedtime routine can be challenging, especially for two-parent households or siblings sharing a room, adding extra logistical considerations.

- **Sleep tips for babies:** Very young babies, lacking a circadian rhythm, may not sleep through the night. If they wake up, try soothing them by talking or touching them without picking them up. Address basic needs like hunger or a diaper change, use minimal lighting, and leave the room calmly.
- **Sleep tips for toddlers:** Young toddlers follow a sleep schedule with daytime napping. Separation anxiety and a fear of missing out can lead to bedtime challenges. Grant them control over minor choices, such as pajamas or bedtime stories. Patience, firmness, and love are crucial to navigating potential power struggles.
- **Sleep tips for school kids:** Busy schedules with academics and extracurricular activities can affect school-age children's sleep. Establish a consistent schedule and a wind-down period before bedtime. Encourage them to do homework or activities outside the bedroom to strengthen the association between the bedroom and sleep.

- **Sleep tips for teenagers:** Teenagers often have a later circadian rhythm, posing challenges with school start times. Acknowledge their busy schedules and collaborate on a healthy sleep routine. Teenagers tend to imitate their parents, so maintaining a healthy sleep pattern yourself is beneficial.

Morning routines matter too. While it's tempting to let kids sleep in on weekends, this can disrupt their sleep schedule. Avoid over-scheduling extracurricular activities if it impacts their sleep. If practicing healthy sleep habits doesn't resolve sleep issues, consulting a doctor or staying informed through the teacher about attention levels may be necessary. Difficulty concentrating, hyperactivity, or learning problems could indicate insufficient sleep.

Sleep Challenges in Children

What may seem trivial to adults can have a profound impact on a child's sleep. Events like the arrival of a new sibling, teething, illnesses, changes in environment or caregivers, alterations in schedules, and minor health issues such as allergies, colds, or ear infections can significantly affect your child's sleep.

Beyond these common challenges, up to 50 percent of children may experience sleep disorders at some point. These disorders are closely linked to both mental and physical health problems, creating a cycle that can be challenging to break. Some sleep disorders may go unnoticed by the sleeper or mimic other conditions like epilepsy, posing difficulties in diagnosis.

Among the prevalent sleep disorders in children are night terrors, nightmares, sleep apnea, sleep talking, sleepwalking, snoring, and restless leg syndrome. Understanding and addressing these issues are crucial for fostering healthy sleep patterns in children.

Nightmares

Nightmares can be unsettling for toddlers, as distinguishing between reality and imagination is challenging for them. These typically occur during REM sleep, leading children to wake up frightened. If this happens, providing reassurance and gently guiding them back to sleep is beneficial.

Night terrors, also known as sleep terrors, are a type of parasomnia that occurs early in the night during non-REM sleep, affecting approximately one-third of children. During a night terror episode, your child may scream and sit up abruptly, but they usually won't fully wake up or recall the incident in the morning. Ensuring your child's safety and attempting to keep them in bed are the primary actions to take. There's typically no need to wake them up, and occasional night terrors are normal. However, if they become frequent or result in daytime sleepiness, it's advisable to discuss them with your pediatrician.

Sleep Talking and Sleepwalking

Sleep talking is a common parasomnia involving verbalization during sleep, often occurring more frequently during lighter sleep phases. Implementing proper sleep hygiene may contribute to reducing sleep-talking episodes. While harmless by itself, sleep talking can be disruptive to others sharing the bedroom. It may also be associated with other sleep disorders like nightmares or sleepwalking.

Research indicates that approximately one in three children will experience sleepwalking before the age of 13, with most incidents happening during the pre-teen years. Similar to sleep talkers, sleepwalkers are unaware of their surroundings and typically have no memory of their actions afterward. Apart from causing daytime sleepiness, sleepwalking can lead to serious consequences based on the individual's activities. If your child experiences sleepwalking, it's advisable to childproof their bedroom and consider installing an alarm. Waking them up approximately half an hour before the expected sleepwalking episode has shown to be beneficial.

Restless Legs Syndrome

Recognized by an irresistible urge to move the legs, identifying restless legs syndrome in children can be challenging. It might initially appear as mere fidgeting or be attributed to growing pains. Managing nighttime restless leg syndrome in children involves implementing proper sleep hygiene and incorporating stretching routines before bedtime. While iron supplements have shown efficacy in treating adults, ongoing research is dedicated to determining the safety and effectiveness of such supplements for children.

If you suspect your child might be dealing with any of these sleep disorders, maintaining a sleep diary to track symptoms and discussing your observations with your pediatrician is a good idea.

Five

Chapter 5 Tips and Tricks and More

Recipes of my Best at home remedies for helping a child stay healthy

The Following are my best tips and tricks for keeping a healthy family and home! All of these are simple and easy to use, some are more geared for older children, and some are really great for smaller children and all are great for adults!

Clean Air in the home:

I use cut-up onions as air filters around my home. what I'll do is I'll chop an onion and half leaving the outer shell of brown skin on it and I place that on my home now what an onion does is when it's cut, it will absorb toxins and germs in the air, leaving behind only the good things Which is why overtime and will get rubbery if it's left out now it'll all absorb whatever environment it's put into so it's best not to store onions in plastic bag because it will absorb the plastic best to only cut onions when you're ready to use them and eat them within a matter of minutes that's one of my tricks that I used to keep my home and air in my house

Another thing I do is I have house plants, which any person who has had house plants and children in the same space knows that's a challenging prospect. It's also very good and there are a few good houseplants you can have around your home that will help your house have clean air and filtered air:

- Spider Plants
- Snake Plants,
- Aloe Vera,
- Parlor Palms,
- Peace Lilies,
- Boston Ferns, to name a few!

House plants are a great addition to any home!

Vitamin C

Another thing I do is make sure my kids get plenty of vitamin C as previously spoken about in this book. There are several ways you can do this of course; eating oranges is a good way but some kids are picky so you gotta get more creative. Kiwis also have very high vitamin C, as well as Pineapples, Strawberries, Papaya, Brussels sprouts, Broccoli, Kale, Parsley, and Cantaloupe.

Foods High in Vitamin C:

- Oranges
- Kiwi's
- Pineapple
- Strawberries
- Papaya
- Brussels Sprouts
- Broccoli
- Kale
- Parsley
- Cantaloupe

You can make homemade vitamin C gummies with orange juice and lemon juice. There are many products out there these days that can provide vitamin C to your child. Gummy ones work best for kids, but some kids don't like the texture so try a couple of options out to see what child your child likes. If you choose to go with the supplement route; best the rule of thumb for vitamin C is that little doses throughout the day are best for your body to utilize the vitamin C.

Daily recommended amount of Vitamin C

Ages 1-3 15 mg per day
  Ages 4-8 25 mg per day
  Ages 9-13 45 mg per day
  Ages 14 and up 65 for girls and 75 for boys

Vitamin C Gummies Recipe at home!

Ingredients:

- 1 1/2 cups orange, cherry, apple or cranberry juice. You can just use one fruit or any combination
- 4 tablespoons plain gelatin
- 2–4 tablespoons raw honey or coconut sugar (use 4 if you like them extra sweet)
- 1/2 teaspoon vanilla extract *optional
- 1 tablespoon Vitamin C powder *optional if you want extra vitamin C

Method:

1. Start by pouring juice into a small saucepan, then sprinkle the gelatin over the top, allowing it to sit for a couple of minutes to "bloom" (you'll notice a wrinkly appearance on the surface). Once the gelatin is absorbed, whisk the mixture to combine.
2. Place the saucepan over medium heat on the stove, ensuring the liquid warms without reaching a boil. Let the gelatin dissolve completely, which typically takes about 3-5 minutes, resulting in a smooth and thin liquid.
3. Introduce honey, and if desired, add vanilla extract and vitamin C powder, mixing well to incorporate all ingredients.
4. Pour the mixture into molds or a loaf pan, then refrigerate for approximately 2-3 hours.
5. Once set, remove the gelatin from the molds. If using a loaf pan, cut the gelatin into small squares for serving.
6. Store these in the refrigerator; they will be good for 2-3

weeks.

Elderberry Syrup

The other great thing I love to do which I always always always have on hand at my home is called elderberry syrup, and this is an amazing tonic, and I make it with water and honey along with several other herbs, which I have the recipe listed in the back of this book or below. Making this with Honey makes it so it's best to give it to older children and adults. Any person of any age can use this tonic it's amazing if you would like to make it for an infant I will put the directions for that below and it will be made with a vegetable glycerin, instead of honey, it will not quite as good as the version made with honey, but it will still give the child the herb infusion that is primarily what we're going forward with this tonic. The dosage for this is variable. As a regular rule of maintenance when your child is healthy, they can be taking 1 tablespoon morning and night or just 1 tablespoon in the morning. When my children are taking this regularly they generally do not catch any of the gunk or sickness that comes home normally from schoolyards. If a child is already sick, you can give them a tablespoon every two hours. No more than 10 tablespoons in 24 hours.

Elderberry Syrup Recipe:

½ cup of Dried Elderberries
5 whole Cloves
1 tablespoon Ginger

1 Cinnamon stick, or 1 Teaspoon ground
2 Cups of Water
1 cup of Honey or vegetable Glycerin (if making for an infant)

Add everything except the Honey into a Medium pot and bring to a boil and simmer for 20 mins, let it cool for 5 mins off the heat, then add the honey, and mix well. At this point, you strain out the Herbs, which you can use a fine mesh strainer or cheese cloth, works well. And it's done! Store in an airtight jar in the fridge for up to 3 months.

Dosage: 1 tablespoon every day for healthy people. 1 table-spoon every two hours when a person is sick.

Honey Garlic Cayenne "HGC"

Another major one that I make is called HGC, which stands for honey garlic cayenne. This is an amazing thing I use for any type of throat or ear infection, sore throat, or an ear infection sinus infection anything of the type. The combination of the honey, the enzymes that come in the raw honey, and also the amazingness of garlic; they're all antiviral to every single one of these ingredients, and the cayenne pepper just gives a boost. Any kind of pepper is going to clean out your system and clear out any kind of infection. It's really really great for attacking those germs that invade your body.

This one's a little bit harder to get little kids to take. They do all right if they can get over a texture and the spiciness, the honey dulls it down some but I do have some members of my family that cannot ingest this remedy. This is a good one for older children who can use mind over matter when it comes to what they can ingest. This is amazing because when I have used it on myself personally, I will take 2-3 teaspoons in the morning and then 1 to 2 teaspoons every two hours throughout the entire day when I'm getting a little bit of sore throat happening and generally every time I have done this the illness goes away by the next morning. It's quite phenomenal and amazing to me. I swear by this remedy it's very helpful and my go-to every time I'm sick; this has been magic for me, and I hope it does for you too!

Honey Garlic Cayenne recipe:

- half a cup of raw Honey,
- 2 tablespoons of chopped garlic
- 2 teaspoons of cayenne pepper.

Mix all together and then store in the fridge for up to 6 weeks.

Dosage: 2 teaspoons, and then 1 teaspoon every 2 hours for 2-3 days depending on the severity of symptoms. Keep using it if your symptoms persist.

Yummy Chicken Noodle Soup

This quick and simple chicken noodle soup serves as an effortless dinner, seamlessly transitioning from stove to table in no time. Utilizing precooked chicken, like rotisserie chicken, expedites the preparation process. With its straightforward and classic ingredients, chicken noodle soup proves to be an excellent introductory dish for discerning eaters.

Ingredients

- 2 Tablespoons Olive Oil
- 2 Large Carrots Sliced thinly
- 3 Stalks Celery Sliced thinly
- 1 Cup Diced Sweet Onion Roughly one medium or half of an extra large onion
- 1 Teaspoon Thyme
- 1 Teaspoon Garlic
- 4 Tablespoons Water
- 1 Teaspoon fresh ginger
- 8 Ounces Egg Noodles This is usually about half of the packs I find at the grocery
- 4 Cups Low Sodium Chicken Broth This is one carton of chicken broth, 32 ounces.
- 2 Cups Cooked Chicken Save time and use rotisserie chicken, cube or shred.
- 4 Cups Water
- 1/2 Teaspoon Salt
- 1/4 Teaspoon Pepper

Instructions

- Add olive oil to the pan and let it warm up. Then add carrots, celery, and onion to the pan and let soften for a minute or two. then add spices and water. Let everything cook for 3-4 minutes. Using an Immersion blender, blend all the veggies together creating a smooth yummy broth.
- Add chicken broth, cooked chicken, dry noodles, and water

to the soup pot. Bring the entire pot to a boil, and cook noodles for the required time on the package. Salt and pepper to taste, and serve!

Nutrition

Calories: 212kcal

Cheesy Broccoli, Chicken and Rice casserole

Ingredients

- ☐ 1 pound chicken breasts cut into chunks
- ☐ 1 teaspoon salt
- ☐ 1 teaspoon pepper
- ☐ 1 teaspoon garlic powder
- ☐ 1 tablespoon olive oil
- ☐ 1 cup white rice
- ☐ 1 cup carrots diced
- ☐ 3 cloves garlic minced
- ☐ 2 1/2 cups chicken stock
- ☐ 2 cups broccoli florets
- ☐ 1 cup grated cheddar

Instructions

1. Season the chicken with salt, pepper, and garlic powder.
2. 1 pound chicken breasts, 1 teaspoon salt, 1 teaspoon pepper, 1 teaspoon garlic powder
3. Add the olive oil to a large, deep skillet and heat until shimmering.
4. 1 tablespoon olive oil
5. Add the chicken to the hot pan and cook, stirring often, until the chicken is nearly cooked through and browned on the outside.
6. Add the rice, carrots, and garlic to the pan and stir to combine. Stir in the chicken broth and bring to a boil.
7. 1 cup white rice, 1 cup carrots, 3 cloves garlic, 2 1/2 cups chicken stock
8. Reduce to a simmer, cover the pan, and cook for 10 minutes.
9. Remove the lid and stir well. Add the broccoli and cover the pan. Continue cooking for 10 minutes or until the liquid has evaporated and the rice is tender.
10. Remove the pan from the heat and sprinkle the cheese on top of the rice mixture. Cover with a lid for 5 minutes to allow the cheese to melt.

Six

Chapter 6 Conclusion

Conclusion

And here we are! This book has been a labor of love for me, and I hope you find these simple tips helpful in your family! I'm by no means done learning, which I will continue to do each day! Life is amazing and full of Glimmers of joy and hope! Look for them!

I find that as I go through life I learn every day. I've learned from all sources of my knowledge of health, From my child's pediatricians, from Holistic sources, learning about how herbs impact the body, and from the words of God! All these things lead to a knowledge of the beautiful body God gave us and as it is my desire to be on God's errand and I hope as I do all the right things that my family will continue to be healthy and that as you ponder this information you'll also find the ones that work for you!

If you found this book helpful, I'd be very appreciative if you'd leave a favorable review for the book on Amazon!

To your health and long life! God Bless!

Warmly, E.A. Keller

Resources

- Campbell, K. (2020, April 22). *Cheesy Chicken and Rice with Broccoli.* Buns in My Oven. Retrieved January 26, 2024, from https://www.bunsinmyoven.com/cheesy-chicken-and-rice/#wprm-recipe-container-26309
- BSc, C. H. M. (2024, January 8). *20 foods that are high in vitamin C.* Healthline. Retrieved January 26, 2024, from https://www.healthline.com/nutrition/vitamin-c-foods#TOC_TITLE_HDR_7
- Care, Y. K. U. (2023, June 14). Vitamin C: the recommended daily dose for kids. *Your Kid's Urgent Care.* Retrieved January 26, 2024, from https://yourkidsurgentcare.com/kids-recommended-daily-dose-of-vitamin-c/
- Creative Healthy Family. (2022, February 24). Homemade Vitamin C Gummies Recipe – Creative Healthy Family. *Creative Healthy Family.* Retrieved January 26, 2024, from https://www.creativehealthyfamily.com/homemade-real-non-gmo-vitamin-c-gummies/

- *default - Stanford Medicine Children's Health.* (n.d.). Retrieved January 26, 2024, from https://www.stanfordchildrens.org/en/topic/default?id=all-about-the-immune-system-90-P01665
- *Home | AAP.* (n.d.). American Academy of Pediatrics. Retrieved January 26, 2024, from https://www.aap.org/
- Kyte Baby. (2021, August 5). Optimal sleep and bedtime windows by age. *Kyte Baby.* Retrieved January 26, 2024, from https://kytebaby.com/blogs/news/optimal-sleep-and-bedtime-windows-by-age
- Pacheco, D., & Pacheco, D. (2023, November 8). *Children and sleep.* Sleep Foundation. Retrieved January 26, 2024, from https://www.sleepfoundation.org/children-and-sleep
- Richardson, K. (2023, September 1). *Super easy chicken noodle soup.* On My Kids Plate. Retrieved January 26, 2024, from https://onmykidsplate.com/easy-chicken-noodle-soup/
- Smallman, E., & Dubuis-Welch, C. (2023, July 3). *These are the best air purifying plants to totally detox your home.* Real Homes. Retrieved January 26, 2024, from https://www.realhomes.com/advice/best-air-purifying-plants
- OpenAI. (n.d.). ChatGPT. Retrieved January 25, 2024, from https://www.openai.com/gpt-3/

Disclaimer

The health advice provided here is for general informational purposes only and should not be considered a substitute for professional medical advice, diagnosis, or treatment. Always seek the advice of your physician or other qualified health provider with any questions you may have regarding a medical condition. Never disregard professional medical advice or delay in seeking it because of content presented. Reliance on any information provided here is solely at your own risk. The contributors and platform disclaim any responsibility for any adverse effects resulting directly or indirectly from the information presented. The information is subject to change or update without notice. Consult a medical professional for personalized health advice tailored to your individual needs and circumstances.

About the Author

E.A. Keller Lives in Northwestern Colorado with her husband and children, where she looks to cook clean meals for her family and make many home remedies to help her family be well! she loves her Chickens and ducks, and the fresh eggs they provide! she enjoys the hillside view out her kitchen window and from her back porch. She enjoys all sorts of games with her family, including board games and video games, she loves to play with Legos and build block towers with her children. She enjoys Cattle work with her husband watching their favorite movies and enjoying audiobooks together!